OSTEOPOROSIS

How to strengthen your *bones*

&

lower your chance of *fracture*

By

William kain

TABLE OF CONTENTS

introduction

Millions of people all around the world are affected by osteoporosis. Loss of bone mass and a higher risk of fractures are its defining traits. Having broken bones is how osteoporosis is understood. Osteoporosis is brought on when the body is unable to keep up with the rate of calcium-related bone mineral loss. When shattered, they become more brittle and lose strength and density. Most people don't realize they have osteoporosis until they break a bone because there aren't many traditional signs or symptoms. The signs and symptoms of osteoporosis, a systemic skeletal disorder, include low bone mass, micro-architectural degradation of bone tissue that results in bone fragility, and an increased risk of fractures. Among the bones that are vulnerable to breaking include the *wrist's bones, the hip joint, and the vertebral column vertebrae.*

Usually, no symptoms exist until a bone is shattered. This book tries to give a thorough analysis of osteoporosis, covering its causes, symptoms, diagnosis, and treatment. The impact of osteoporosis on one's quality of life as well as the numerous methods for managing and preventing this condition will also be covered.

Chapter 1

Osteoporosis

*The term "osteoporosis" and its frequency

A decline in bone density and quality, which raises the risk of fractures, is the hallmark of the medical disorder osteoporosis. It is a prevalent condition that primarily **affects elderly women**, however, it can also **affect younger people**. Osteoporosis develops when bones lose calcium and other minerals more quickly than the body can replenish them. This causes bones to weaken, become brittle, and become more prone to breaking, especially in the wrist, hip, and spine. *An osteoporotic fracture occurs in one in three women over 50 and one in five men over 50, according to the International Osteoporosis Foundation, which estimates that osteoporosis affects 200 million people globally.* Because of the high morbidity, mortality, and financial costs related to fractures, it is a significant health concern. Early diagnosis, prevention, and treatment are therefore crucial for controlling osteoporosis.

*Osteoporosis and Inflammation

Bone loss can result from chronic systemic inflammation in a variety of different ways. Cytokines are molecular messengers that alert immune cells to move to an infection or injury location. **Cytokines** are produced as a result of **inflammation**. The activity of cells called osteoclasts, which are in charge of destroying bone tissue, can be stimulated by certain of these cytokines, including *TNF-alpha and IL-1*. Osteoporosis risk can rise as a result, and bone density can be lost. *The harmony between bone growth and bone resorption can also be thrown off by persistent inflammation. Bone tissue normally* *undergoes a process called remodeling in which it is continually destroyed and replaced.* This process can be hampered by inflammation, which eventually causes a net loss of bone. In addition, osteoblasts, which are responsible for forming new bone tissue, can have their function affected by chronic inflammation. By doing so, the loss of bone density may worsen even more, raising the possibility of fractures. *Overall, persistent systemic inflammation can negatively affect bone health, so inflammation control is essential for preserving bone strength and health.*

*gastrointestinal system and osteoporosis

Osteoporosis is a disease of the bones that weakens and brutalizes them, increasing the risk of fractures. *Although osteoporosis predominantly affects the skeletal system,* it can also impact other body systems, such as the digestive system. Osteoporosis may reduce the amount of bone in the spine's vertebrae, which may have an impact on the digestive system. Osteoporosis weakens the vertebrae, which can lead to their collapsing and compressing of the spinal cord's nerves. Constipation, bloating, and discomfort in the abdomen may result from this. Additionally, some osteoporosis drugs, such as bisphosphonates, can have adverse digestive side effects including *nausea, vomiting, and stomach pain.* These drugs function by delaying the deterioration of bone tissue, which can result in an accumulation of calcium in the blood and raise the risk of kidney stones. Even while osteoporosis mostly affects the skeletal system, it can also have effects on the digestive system, especially when the spine's vertebrae are involved or when drugs are used to treat the illness. *It's vital to speak with your healthcare professional if you are worried about how osteoporosis may be impacting your digestive system.*

Chapter 2

*Risk factors and causes of osteoporosis

Osteoporosis can occur for some reasons and have several risk factors.

(Age) Osteoporosis risk can be increased as we age since our bones become less thick and more brittle.

(Gender) After menopause, osteoporosis is more common in women than in males.

(Family history) If a close relative suffers from osteoporosis, your risk of getting it yourself may be higher.

(Unbalanced hormones) Having low amounts of testosterone in men and estrogen in women can make you more likely to develop osteoporosis.

(Unhealthy diet) An osteoporosis risk-raising diet includes calcium and vitamin D deficiencies.

(Living a sedentary lifestyle) Bone thinning and osteoporosis risk are both increased by inactivity and prolonged sitting.

(Smoking) By lowering bone density, smoking can raise the risk of osteoporosis.

(Alcohol abuse) Drinking too much alcohol can weaken bones and increase the chance of fractures.

(Conditions) several illnesses, including *celiac disease,*

inflammatory bowel disease, and *several cancers*, can raise the risk of osteoporosis.

(*Drugs*) Long-term use of some drugs, including *corticosteroids and anticonvulsants*, can raise the risk of osteoporosis.

It's crucial to keep in mind that a combination of these variables frequently leads to osteoporosis, and some people may be more prone to the ailment than others. Consult your doctor if you have any concerns about your risk of developing osteoporosis

*chemicals in the environment and bone loss

Toxins from the environment can harm bone health and accelerate bone thinning. Heavy metals including lead and cadmium, insecticides, and air pollution are some of the most prevalent environmental pollutants that have been connected to bone loss. By interfering with the development of new bone tissue and upsetting the balance of minerals like calcium and phosphorus in the bones, lead, for instance, might hinder the body's capacity to develop and maintain strong bones. Another heavy metal, cadmium, has been associated with a rise in fracture risk, particularly in females, as well as a reduction in bone density.

Additionally demonstrated to have detrimental impacts on bone health are pesticides. *It has been proven that exposure to several pesticides, including pyrethroids and organophosphates, lowers bone density and increases the risk of fractures.* Bone loss has also been linked to air pollution, particularly fine particulate matter (PM2.5). It has been demonstrated that prolonged exposure to high PM2.5 levels reduces bone density and raises the risk of osteoporosis. Overall, limiting one's exposure to environmental contaminants is crucial for maintaining bone health. Avoiding exposure to pesticides and heavy metals, utilizing air purifiers to lessen indoor air pollution, and supporting laws that support clean air and water are some ways to achieve this. In addition, leading a healthy lifestyle that includes regular exercise and calcium- and vitamin D-rich, balanced diet will help safeguard bone health.

*Osteoporosis and hormonal factors.

Osteoporosis is a disorder marked by a gradual decrease in bone mass and density, which raises the fragility and fracture risk. In controlling bone metabolism and the onset of osteoporosis, hormones are essential. *Estrogen is a crucial hormone in the metabolism of bones.* In premenopausal women, estrogen is predominantly produced by the ovaries, and it aids in promoting bone growth and preventing bone resorption. There is a net loss of bone mass and density after menopause when estrogen levels fall and bone resorption outpaces bone synthesis. *The hormone parathyroid is another hormone that affects bone metabolism. (PTH).*

The production of PTH by the parathyroid glands aids in controlling blood calcium levels. When blood calcium levels are low, PTH encourages the release of calcium from bone, which can eventually cause bone loss. PTH can aid to drive bone production and boost bone density when it is released sporadically, though. The hormone calcitonin also controls the metabolism of bones. It is made by the thyroid gland and aids in preventing bone loss so that bone density is preserved.

Hormones are essential for controlling osteoporosis development and bone metabolism. While PTH and calcitonin assist in controlling blood calcium levels and preserving bone density, estrogen aids in bone growth and inhibits bone resorption. These hormone imbalances have been linked to osteoporosis development and bone loss.

*Osteoporosis symptoms and signs
Reduced bone density and strength are symptoms of osteoporosis, which increases the risk of fractures. *Among the*

symptoms of osteoporosis are the following:

*backache

*height decline with time

*hunched position

*bone fractures that happen more frequently than anticipated, particularly in the wrist, hip, or spine

*reduced grip power in the arm

*a weakened state of the muscles encircling the injured bones

stiffness or joint discomfort

tooth loss as the supporting bones for the teeth deteriorate

Vertebral compression fractures can cause spinal abnormalities or potentially compress the spinal cord in extreme circumstances.

It is crucial to speak with your doctor if you are experiencing any of these signs or are worried about your risk for osteoporosis. *To assist you manage your disease, they can suggest diagnostic procedures and possible courses of therapy.*

Chapter 3

Osteoporosis Diagnosis

*screening for osteoporosis

There are numerous ways to check for osteoporosis, including.

The most frequent test to identify osteoporosis is (**dual-energy X-ray absorptiometry (DXA)** At the hip, spine, and other skeletal locations, it measures bone density using a low-dose X-ray.

(**Quantitative computed tomography (QCT)** This test makes use of a CT scanner to assess the spine's and the hip's bone density. The measurement of bone density is more precise than with DXA, but it is more expensive.

(*Peripheral dual-energy X-ray*) absorptiometry (pDXA) is a test that analyzes bone density in the wrist, heel, or finger. It is similar *to DXA*.

(*Ultrasound*) This examination measures the density of the bone at the heel, shinbone, and kneecap. Although less expensive than **DXA**, it could not be as precise.

(**Biochemical indicators of bone turnover**)These examinations look for specific substances in the blood or urine that show how quickly bones are degraded and regenerated. They are not used to identify osteoporosis, but they can be useful in assessing how well a treatment is working. As well as younger people with certain risk factors like low body weight, a family history of osteoporosis, or a history of fractures, it is advised that men and women over the age of 70 and 65, respectively, undergo screenings for osteoporosis.

*Results of bone density tests are interpreted

To identify osteoporosis or determine a person's risk of getting the condition, bone density tests are frequently utilized. A T-score or a Z-score is used to describe a bone density test's outcomes.

The T-score contrasts the bone density of a person with the typical bone density of a healthy young adult of the same sex. Normal bone density is defined as a T-score of -1.0 or higher. Low bone density or osteopenia, which may increase the risk of fracture, is indicated by a T-score between -1.0 and -2.5. Osteoporosis, which considerably raises the risk of fracture, is indicated by a T-score of -2.5 or lower.

A person's bone density is compared using the Z-score to the average bone density of people their age, sex, and body size. Further testing might be required if the Z-score is -2.0 or lower, raising concerns. It's crucial to remember that other factors, like age, family history, and lifestyle choices, may also affect an individual's risk of fracture and outweigh the impact that bone density tests play in this regard. It is crucial to speak with your healthcare practitioner if you have any queries or concerns regarding the findings of your bone density test. They can answer your questions and, if necessary, prescribe the best course of action.

*Additional osteoporosis diagnostic tests

There are several diagnostic methods than bone mineral density (BMD) testing that can be used to detect osteoporosis or gauge the risk of fractures:

(Vertebral Fracture Assessment (VFA) is an X-ray imaging method that focuses on searching for fractures in the spine's bones. Vertebral fractures that may not be seen on standard X-rays can be found using VFA.

(Quantitative Ultrasound (QUS) This non-invasive test measures the density of the bones in the heel, shinbone, or finger by using sound waves. It is a portable,

affordable test that can be used to check for osteoporosis in huge populations.

(*Lab tests*) Calcium, phosphate, vitamin D, and other hormone levels that may have an impact on bone health can be assessed using blood tests. With the aid of these tests, the underlying causes of bone loss can be found or other conditions that may resemble osteoporosis can be ruled out.

(*FRAX (Fracture Risk Assessment Tool*) Based on risk factors like age, sex, body mass index (BMI), prior fractures, family history, and lifestyle choices, FRAX calculates a person's 10-year probability of suffering a hip fracture or a major osteoporotic fracture. It's crucial to remember that these diagnostic tests are used in conjunction with a medical history, physical examination, and other risk factors to establish a person's overall risk of developing osteoporosis and fractures rather than being used alone to diagnose osteoporosis.

Chapter 4

Osteoporosis Treatment

*Lifestyle modifications

Osteoporosis is a disorder in which the loss of bone density causes the bones to become thin and brittle. Several dietary adjustments can help manage or prevent osteoporosis, including *Strength and bone density can be enhanced with regular exercise, particularly weight-bearing activities. Walking, jogging, dancing, and weightlifting are a few examples of weight-bearing exercises.* The health of your bones depends on calcium, vitamin D, and K2. Taking vitamin D pills and eating calcium-rich foods like milk, cheese, yogurt, and leafy greens can help increase bone density. Smoking has been associated with an increased risk of osteoporosis because it can cause bone loss. *Smoking* cessation can enhance bone density and general health. Overindulging in alcohol can result in bone loss and raise the risk of fractures. To preserve bone health, alcohol use should be kept to a minimum. *Falls and fractures* are made more likely by osteoporosis. *Fractures can be prevented by taking preventative measures such as building grab bars, using non-slip mats, and dressing appropriately.* Individuals can improve their overall bone health and reduce their risk of fractures by implementing these lifestyle changes to help prevent or manage osteoporosis.

*Relation Between Osteoporosis & Arthritis

While osteoporosis is a disorder that affects the bones, arthritis, and osteoarthritis are two conditions that affect the joints. Despite being separate situations, there is some overlap in the ways that they might influence one another. A range of diseases collectively referred to as arthritis induces inflammation in the joints. Rheumatoid arthritis and osteoarthritis are the two most prevalent kinds of arthritis. Osteoarthritis is degenerative if they use corticosteroids to treat their arthritic symptoms. This is due to the possibility that corticosteroids may eventually cause the bones to weaken. Similarly to this, individuals with osteoarthritis may have a higher chance of getting osteoporosis, especially if their mobility is restricted and they are less active due to their joint discomfort. *This is because maintaining bone density requires weight-bearing activity, and individuals with osteoarthritis may be less inclined to do so if they are experiencing joint discomfort. In conclusion, although osteoporosis and arthritis are separate diseases, there are a variety of ways in which they are connected.* People who have arthritis, especially rheumatoid arthritis, may be more likely to develop osteoporosis, whereas those who have osteoarthritis may be more likely to do so if their joint discomfort prevents them from being as active.

Chapter 5

*Foods & Nutrients for osteoporosis

Broken bones, also known as fractures, can happen as a result of trauma, falls, or repeated stress on the bones. Fractures are treated differently depending on where, how severe, and what kind of fracture they are. *Immobilization* For the broken bone to heal properly, this entails keeping it in a fixed position. Casts, splints, or braces

can be used to achieve immobility.
Medications The discomfort brought on by fractures might be lessened by using painkillers. *Surgery* could be required in some circumstances to straighten and stabilize the shattered bone. This is especially true for fractures involving joint surfaces or complicated fractures. *Physical therapy* can aid in regaining the damaged area's strength, flexibility, and range of motion once the fracture has healed. electrical arousal To promote

bone repair during this procedure, low-level electrical currents are used. nutritional assistance Calcium, vitamin D, and other nutrients must be consumed in sufficient amounts to promote bone health and the healing process. For guidance on the ideal fracture treatment strategy, speak with a healthcare expert.

*Vitamin and mineral contributions to osteoporosis

Maintaining bone health and avoiding osteoporosis require vitamins and minerals. Bones that have osteoporosis are weak and brittle, which makes them more prone to breaking. The following essential vitamins and minerals are crucial for avoiding osteoporosis:

(Calcium) Calcium is necessary for the development and maintenance of strong bones. Calcium is

necessary for the body to produce bones and teeth, as well as for muscular contraction, nerve signaling, and blood coagulation. Dairy products, leafy green vegetables, and fortified foods are examples of foods high in calcium.

(Vitamin D) Vital for healthy bones, vitamin D aids in the body's absorption of calcium. Additionally, it affects the immune system, muscles, and cell development. Sunlight is the

finest source of vitamin D, although it can also be found in fatty fish, egg yolks, and foods that have been fortified.

(**Magnesium**) Magnesium aids in bone development and controls the body's calcium levels. *Additionally, it affects how muscles, nerves, and the metabolism of energy work. Nuts, seeds, whole grains, and leafy green vegetables* are among the foods high in magnesium.

(Vitamin K) Vitamin K supports bone health and aids in calcium regulation. *Additionally, it aids in blood coagulation and might be anti-inflammatory. Cheese, egg yolks, soybeans, broccoli, and leafy green vegetables all contain vitamin K.*

(Zinc) Zinc aids in the body's use of calcium and is crucial for bone development. *Additionally, it affects protein synthesis, wound healing, and immunological function.*

Meat, shellfish, nuts, and seeds are among the foods high in zinc.

*(**Vitamin C**)* Collagen, a crucial component of bone tissue, is synthesized with the help of vitamin C. *Additionally, it aids in immunological function and has antioxidant characteristics. Citrus fruits, berries, and peppers are particularly high in vitamin C, as are other fruits and vegetables.*

* vitamin **K2's** role in the treatment of osteoporosis

Maintaining bone health and preventing osteoporosis are major functions of *vitamin K2.* The illness known as osteoporosis is defined by a decline in bone density, which raises the risk of fractures. The *protein osteocalcin*, which is crucial for the development of bones, is activated by *vitamin K2.* By aiding in the *binding of calcium* and *other minerals* to the

bone matrix, osteocalcin helps to strengthen and increase the fracture resistance of bones. Furthermore, *vitamin K2 has been demonstrated to aid in preventing the loss of calcium from bones.* This is significant since calcium is a crucial component of bone tissue and a deficiency could result in weakening bones. Numerous studies have revealed that vitamin K2 supplements can increase bone density and lower fracture risk in both men and women. Women who took a daily vitamin K2 supplement, for instance, had a considerably lower incidence of hip fractures than those who did not, according to one study. Overall, vitamin K2 is crucial for maintaining bone strength and preventing osteoporosis. It's crucial to make sure that you get enough of this vitamin through a balanced diet or supplements, especially if you're at risk for osteoporosis. In general, a well-balanced diet rich in essential vitamins and minerals, regular exercise, abstaining from smoking and excessive alcohol consumption, and eating a balanced diet will help prevent osteoporosis and maintain bone health.

*foods to consume for a stronger bone system

Numerous foods can support healthier bones overall and stronger bones in particular. Calcium is abundant in milk, cheese, and yogurt and is crucial for the health of the bones. The *calcium* and other *minerals* that are excellent for the bones, such as *vitamin K*, can be found in *leafy green vegetables like kale, spinach, and collard greens.* **Salmon** The body may more easily absorb calcium because of this fish's high vitamin D content. *Calcium and vitamin D* are often added as food additives to items like cereal and orange juice, Calcium can be found in nuts and seeds including sesame, chia, and almonds. *The minerals* that support bone health are abundant in beans and legumes like lentils, chickpeas, and kidney beans. Calcium, magnesium, and phosphorus are abundant components in *bone broth*, which is also produced by *simmering animal bones and connective tissue*. To construct and maintain strong bones, it's crucial to eat a balanced diet as well as to exercise that involves bearing weight, such as walking or weightlifting.

In conclusion

*Osteoporosis-fighting Anabolic Body

Due to its ability to strengthen bones and increase bone density, anabolic bodybuilding can be helpful for people with osteoporosis. You can take the following actions to build an anabolic physique and lower your risk of osteoporosis:

Strengthen your muscles and bones by including resistance training exercises in your workout routine, such as weightlifting or the use of resistance bands. Resistance exercise is essential for maintaining muscle mass and increasing bone density, both of which are necessary for preventing osteoporosis.

Consume a well-balanced meal that contains enough protein, carbs, and good fats. While carbs give energy for workouts and healthy fats are crucial for hormone production and overall health, a sufficient protein intake is required to create and maintain muscle mass.

To obtain these nutrients, include foods high in calcium, vitamin D, and vitamin K2 in one meal or supplement. Calcium helps to strengthen bones while vitamin D facilitates calcium absorption. And vitamin K2 sends the calcium's final product directly to the bone rather than the artery. Excellent sources of calcium include dairy products, leafy greens, and meals that have been fortified. Vitamin D is found in fatty fish, eggs, and fortified meals, but it can also be obtained via sunlight, *(K2) mk4 and mk7* are necessary for the production of bones, even though vitamin K2 comes from the fermented natto product.

(Rest and recovery) Give yourself enough time to recover and rest

between workouts to avoid overuse injuries and encourage muscle growth. Rest days are crucial for muscular growth, and your body needs time to recuperate and repair after a hard workout.

Consult a medical professional: If you have osteoporosis, you should speak with a medical professional before beginning a new exercise regimen or making nutritional adjustments. They can provide you with advice on safe and efficient workouts and suggest any dietary changes that are required.

References about osteoporosis

In her early 35s, my wife was found to have osteopenia despite having healthy, vibrant bones. She was diagonal with osteoporosis and the cause of her bone loss was discovered. After that, we began looking for natural ways to promote her health. We began taking all the necessary precautions about her diet, and fitness and making sure she never lacks all the important vitamins & minerals that are essential for bone formation. *Now that osteoporosis has been identified, researchers can work to prevent it.* To help us get a head start on the road to bone building, we conduct several research investigations. Losing bones is not a given. Our food doesn't include enough of the nutrients that healthy bones require, which is an issue. *Osteoporosis can be caused by a combination of factors, including common chemicals, heavy metals, and other pollutants found in our environment.* The good news is that you may avoid or decrease the effects of every single one of these bone-crunching factors. Simple methods for bone healing are revealed. The specific nutrients, many of which are lacking in ordinary meals, that our bones require, from vitamin A to zinc and from vitamin D and K2. *(Studies show most of us are deficient in at least some of these.)* If despite your best efforts, you are still losing bone. Learn about the lab tests that can tell you how vitamin-rich you are and how to overcome genetic disadvantages. The fantastic part is right here. Bone health is beneficial to your overall health! *It is made to aid in bone growth and strengthening,* but there are many other advantages.

For your bones to remain strong and healthy, they need a variety of nutrition, little exposure to dangerous substances, and weight-bearing exercise. You are definitely on your path to eventually beating osteoporosis if you adhere to the tips offered here for building healthy bones. It's important to take medications as directed by your doctor if you want to slow bone loss and lower your risk of fractures. *Discuss fall prevention with your doctor. Talking with your doctor about fall prevention strategies, such as clearing your house of dangers, utilizing assistive technology, and enhancing balance, is vital because falls can result in fractures* The best course of action for you will depend on how well you stay informed about the most recent findings in osteoporosis research and treatment options. Remember that managing osteoporosis early on can help prevent problems and enhance the overall quality of life. Take preventative measures to control osteoporosis and safeguard your bone health if you are at risk for it or have been diagnosed with it.

www.ingramcontent.com/pod-product-compliance
Lightning Source LLC
Chambersburg PA
CBHW071046220526
45467CB00004B/1690